Beating Alzheimer's

Life-Altering Tips to Help Prevent You from Becoming Another Statistic

This book is dedicated to Bob and Marge Tuttle. May your love for each other transcend the chord of this life.

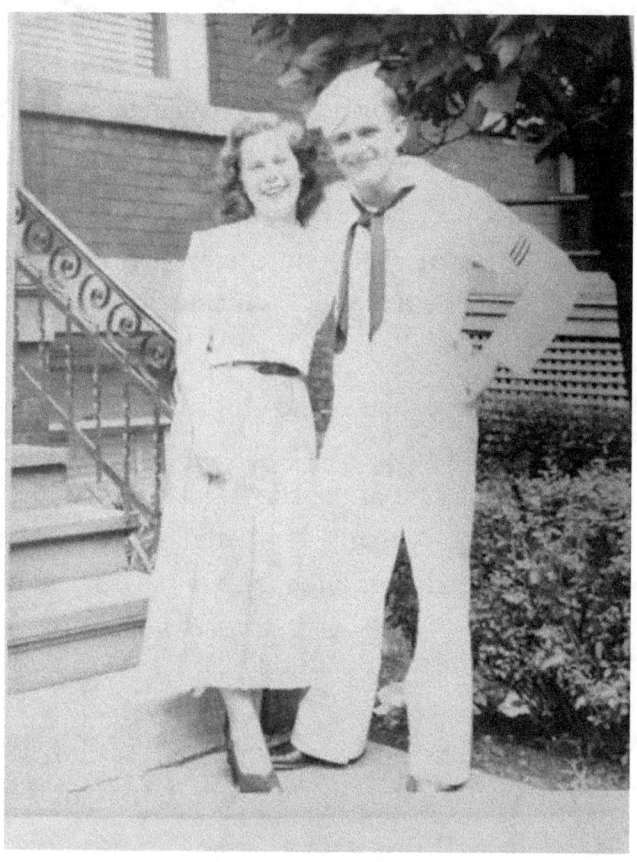

Table of Contents

Preface

"There ain't no atheists in a foxhole!"

Now there's a statement to make you stop and think about life's priorities. I remember an old Marine, a Korean War Veteran, made that several statement years ago. Over the years, my mind would let it come and go for reasons beyond my comprehension. However, one fact remains; it has stuck with me as if he just said it.

In the late 1980's, and into the early 1990's, I spent the better part of five years practicing digging foxholes. In my years as a U.S. Army Military Police Officer, I would work two weeks patrolling the streets of the Army base and two weeks working on field drills.

In those days, we trained in the German woods with the anticipation of war against communist countries. Foxholes where very much a part of our field training.

In the field, once we established where to set up camp, each soldier dug a foxhole to form an outer perimeter around camp. Our tool of the trade was an Army-issued shovel called an E-Tool. As we sat in our foxholes, our job was to protect the brass (our fearless leaders) and equipment.

It wasn't uncommon that we'd joke about using these tiny shovels to dig our own grave. The military has a knack for bringing out a unique sense of humor in a person. Later I learned it was our individualized coping mechanisms: A way to put up (and accept) with the stress.

Now let's go back to the opening statement. *"There ain't no atheists in a foxhole!"*

Over the years I've looked at the meaning of this profound statement from just about every angle. And my years of wisdom has led to this conclusion.

Imagine standing neck-deep in your own foxhole. The enemy is throwing a constant barrage of rounds your way with one intention: To kill you. Then, take your position. With your life at its possible end – in between dodging bullets and the screams from the guys in the foxholes around you – you pray.

Praying to our creator, God.

Every one of us will find ourselves sitting in that proverbial foxhole at some point in our life. Many won't know it until right before it happens, but others will see it coming.

Call it fortune or misfortune; nevertheless, it is a fact.

Every one of us will find ourselves sitting in that proverbial foxhole at some point in our life. Many won't know it until right before it happens, but others will see it coming.

Call it fortune or misfortune; nevertheless, it is a fact.

The reason for writing this book is simple. Lately there had been a tugging, no more like a *calling* on my heart (and life) and it's been active for a while now. But it wasn't until just before sitting down to write this book did it make sense.

If I thought about it hard and long enough, I would say it was after hearing the words of the song, *Start a Fire* by the band Unspoken. I would focus on the lyrics every time the song came on the radio. It started to resonate deep in my soul.

These stories – and this calling – come together as I start to understand that God has started a fire in me to help create bigger change in this world. Not in a generic, *"I want to help people"* fashion. It goes MUCH deeper than that.

As the story unfolds, you will learn about a man who I've only known for a few years, but his impact upon me will last a life-time. This man–

Robert Tuttle, raised nine children, many of whom he scared the life out of more than a few times as they grew up.

For example, on family trips Bob would pass cars on the right shoulder if they were driving too slow. It didn't matter if the road was two or four lanes, he would pass them on the right shoulder.

To this day I get a kick out of listening to each of the kids tell the story from their own perspectives. One common thread was he'd race past the violating driver holding his koozie out the driver's side window. The real kicker, the koozie had a County Sheriff's Star on it (like a police badge). And of course there would be a can of Blatz beer inside. As he passed other drivers, doing something "stupid," he waved the beer-loaded koozie to get their attention and to straighten up.

You can't make this stuff up!

As God's grace would have it, one of his nine children, Carole, became my lovely wife in 2011. She is the youngest of the crew. Since meeting her, I've come to know her dad Bob, or better known as Poppie. Every time we would drive to Fort Wayne to visit him, he would tell me about his days in the Navy. He had great stories; even if I did hear the same ones every time we visited.

When we arrived home, he would always shake my hand and try to squeeze it as hard as he could. *"I still got it"* would follow every handshake. When it was time to leave, he would give me a hug and squeeze just as hard as he did with his handshake.

Again, *"I still got it!"* would ring from his lips along with his notorious mischievous smile.

As you partake in this man's journey, understand the calling placed on my heart. My goal is to help you learn more about this devastating disease – Alzheimer's. Many Americans believe Alzheimer's is a natural part of growing old. What is more startling is many are under the impression they will get it, too.

I hope to shed some light on this still little-known disease with the following words, as well as provide tools to help your loved-one who may be sitting in their proverbial "foxhole."

Introduction

No matter how hard I try, the words to describe my frustration with Alzheimer's Disease stays just out of reach. Just like the elusive trophy-fish that jumps out of your hands as you reel it onto the boat, understanding this disease is enough to make one jump into a river.

All of the needless suffering, the pointless pain for those with loved ones suffering from the deadly disease can be frustrating. As I put pen to paper to write this book, I constantly come across media posts that cause me to question my decision.

There are numerous examples of people who live *healthy* and develop the disease. After years in health and fitness, my only conclusion is one person's definition of healthy is not the best definition: Nor the only definition.

Sit down and turn on your television, radio, or walk into any gym around the world, and you will notice one thing; no two resources will have the same "secret sauce" for optimal health.

I've been asked the same question a thousand times. *"What works?"*

My answer, *"Everything, to an extent."*

What works for you may or may not work for someone else. Any change you make will facilitate a different path in your life. Depending on your why for the change will determine its sticking ability. When you refuse to make a change (from your current course), you open yourself up to becoming what I call The Walking Sick. This is where the pre-disease lingers.

While I write these exact words, family members have decided against putting a feeding tube in Bob. I've done enough research to know most people eventually pass-away from Alzheimer's due to their loss of appetite. The human body starts to shut down without proper nourishment and hydration.

It's hard not to think about how the next (and final) stage of the disease is just around the corner. Bringing me back to the reason why I decided to stick with writing this book.

Too many people needlessly let their lives pass them by. So many of us, including myself, spend countless hours wishing we did more with our precious time. The problem is we make that wish at the most inopportune times. Then, one day, as if it snuck up on us, we can't remember the person sitting across from us. Memories, thoughts, dreams, and goals fade fast. And in the latter stages it's almost by the minute.

It's at this time in our lives the events of yesterday turn into a distant memory, soon to be lost in the depths of our dying neurons.

Robert Tuttle, though you may never get a chance to read this book, you are the inspiration for these words. I finally got up and decided to make some type of change in this world because of you, by offering ways to help beat Alzheimer's through prevention.

Countless people lose their lives every day due to a form of dementia, specifically Alzheimer's. Year after year money is raised, events are promoted, and people participate in some type of fundraising activity to help find a cure. But the cause, let alone the cure remain elusive.

This book has been broken down into two sections with a special section of stories the family wanted to share about Poppie.

Section One:

This section describes Alzheimer's, how it happens, how to identify the symptoms, and what to do if you believe you or a loved one is progressing through the initial stages of the disease.

Section Two:

This section will give you subtle life-style changes you can make every day to help slow down the progression and perhaps prevent the disease. I will give you exercises, nutrition tips, and resources to help you flex your brain muscle.

The one question constantly nagging me: "Why isn't more emphasis placed on prevention. I understand, just as with every other disease, there _is_ a need for treating the disease. We all strive for the best of what life has to offer. What we need, however, is more emphasis on prevention. Is it because you won't find billions of dollars in profit by preventing the disease? Or, are there other contributing factors (people) keeping prevention at arm's length?

My goal is to help you avoid Alzheimer's; to help you prevent it from taking over your life. Whether directly or indirectly through family or friends, if I can help one person NOT get Alzheimer's, then I've accomplished what I set out to do.

What You Can Expect From This Book

At the beginning of each Chapter, I provide a short story about Poppie the family decided to share with the world. Though Alzheimer's is a serious disease, there are times you can still enjoy as the disease progresses. We all have a story and our lives are ever evolving.

It's all about perception. You can look at it in a way that causes depression, but honestly, no one wants to be around someone like that. Make the remaining time with your loved ones fun, joyous, and continue to make new memories.

Within these pages, I will provide you a definitive action plan. A plan showing you subtle life style changes you can easily accomplish, without drastically changing your life.

There is only one thing I ask. Take this information and apply it!

It is that simple. Far too many people will buy into a solution and not act on what they learn. Even the smallest of forward momentum will get you traveling in the right direction.

The question is, *"Are you ready – and willing – to take that first step?"*

When I first sat down to write this book I had to answer this one question; *"Who am I to be considered an authority on a topic degreed researchers have a hard time describing, preventing, or curing?"*

Honestly, I'm confident in my answer to that question. The human body is a remarkable specimen. I understand what people can do to improve their chances at reversing life threatening ailments through proper nutrition, exercise, and simple lifestyle habits.

One of the biggest roadblocks I suffer from – whether self-imposed or legitimate – is the fact that my prevention measures may never prove to be effective. Before you put this book down, let me explain.

One of the biggest reasons why big pharma doesn't want anything to do with prevention is: At this point in the game it's next to impossible to track whether it is working or not. It's much easier to research and distribute medications that, at best, mask the issue at hand.

Prevention is an ugly term to those types of companies. Really, how can you track prevention? Either you get the disease or you don't. Unless you get a large group of volunteers who are willing to participate for a big chunk of their lives, tracking will be next to impossible.

But, if I can help one person live a healthier life and never have to fight off a disease, then I have succeeded. It's about giving you the tools to bring out the best of your life.

When you break down the basics, none of it is really rocket science. It's all about knowing what to do and more importantly, taking the steps and doing it. One of the biggest roadblocks associated with being a Fitness Professional is the lack of action in many of the people who seek me out. They seem to resist action as if it was some type of plague.

How do I know? Because I'm the same way. Well, except for exercise and nutrition.

Learning new things can be exciting. No matter if it's a book, a Podcast, or a lecture on a topic that excites you, learning can be rewarding. However, when the learning portion is over, with every passing second, your chances of success dwindle the longer you wait to act.

There is NEVER a perfect time, nor with there ever be one.

As you progress through this book, be open to the techniques you will learn. Embrace them with open arms. Accept them as a part of your life. In addition, teach others to do them as well. The more people you bring into your circle, the more lives you can affect.

Once you practice these techniques, every aspect of your life will start to change. I encourage you to take action; even if it is one tip here and another tip there. Alzheimer's is a disease with the potential of becoming a pandemic. It knows no boundaries and has no prejudice.

What it does have is the ability to steal your dreams, your memories, your thoughts, and the life you once knew.

"The future depends on what you do today."

— **Mahatma Gandhi**

Section I

Alzheimer's – The Past, Present & Future

Be still, and know that I am God – Psalms 46:10

Chapter 1

The second you stop learning is the second you start dying. – ***Author unknown***

The Day I Couldn't Remember....

It was a sunny mid-summer day in December. I find myself standing here in my kitchen, gazing, dreaming while peering out the window. My thoughts seem to escape me right now. I know I was thinking about something. Maybe it is just a way for me to get lost in my thoughts, thinking about nothing in particular – almost a form of standing meditation.

The sun is shining bright on this Sunday afternoon. It is the time between fall and winter and can bring crazy weather. Nonetheless, I see the squirrels running around the back yard chasing each other – frolicking in a way only squirrels can do.

I think to myself, "I'm sure they're playing, or maybe fighting over the last of the fall feast spread out over the yard." They're taking full advantage of each minute of daylight; these are the last few days before our Indiana winter sets in.

My baby girl (and her husband) are here making lunch for mom and me. Every Sunday one of the kids visits and makes us lunch. This is a time to enjoy family and to eat some good food.

I break out of my meditative trance. I look over my left shoulder and see Carole (my baby girl) at the kitchen counter cutting fresh veggies. I instantly break free of my empty thoughts, look down, and see I'm standing in front of the dish drainer. I notice a few dishes needing to be tended to and commence to putting them away.

Aaah...here we go...my cereal bowl. I'll take this and put it away.

As I pick it up, it occurs to me I'm not sure where it goes. Standing here in front of the cabinet, I look at this small plastic blue object and

11

concentrate on where it's suppose to go. I'm sure if anyone was watching me I'd resemble an alien (from one of those classic cheesy sci-fi movies) trying to figure out what this *foreign* earth object was.

Hold on...wait a minute...it's almost there...

I look up at cabinet that is staring back at me. Then I look down at the bowl, then back at the cabinet one more time.

"Nope! It doesn't go there," I say to myself.

I do a 180 and look over to the other side of the kitchen. *I'll head over by the stove and get this thing put away once and for all.*

Okay, where does thing go again? Maybe it goes in the top shelf of this big white cabinet next to the stove. I take another glance at the bowl, look back up at the cabinet and reach for the handle to open the door.

With my left hand, I grab the handle to pull it open. It suddenly occurs to me this cabinet seems to be colder than I remembered.

In one swift pull, the door opens to my left and out rushes a blast of freezing air.

Why would this cabinet be so cold?

I again look down at the blue object in my hand, back up at what happens to be the freezer and mouth the word, "D@mmit!" In a little fit of frustration, I close the freezer door, turn back to the dish drainer and place the bowl back where I found it. I then notice the beautiful sun shining outside as the squirrels play...*Hey, maybe I should put this bowl away.*

This, my friends, is only a snippet of the life of someone living with Alzheimer's. One mere moment in a day riddled with forgetting what was once the obvious. Though I added a few details about this story, everything Poppie did was what I observed while sitting at the kitchen table on that particular Sunday.

12

Sometimes we joke about what it would be like to start over each day, just as someone living with Alzheimer's has to do. Not by choice, but because of the cards they've been dealt. In reality, this is not something <u>anyone</u> deserves, let alone wants to live with.

Try to imagine the frustration of not being able to recall the simple things in life. The stress it causes and the grief; not only for the person suffering from it, but family and friends who are involved.

Though there are several contributing factors to this disease, often referred to as Type 3 Diabetes (or Diabetes of the brain), there are things you can do to help prevent this disease from taking root in your own health.

In my research, there were three important factors proving the most beneficial in prevention:

1. Nutrition

2. Exercise

3. Brain Strength (Health)

You have heard it before and will hear it repeatedly. Change the way you eat, increase your activity level, and flex your brain muscle. As you become increasingly intentional with nutrition, exercise, and working on mental strength, your chances of developing Alzheimer's drops drastically. (Not to mention decreased chances of developing several other inflammatory issues.)

More simplistically, eat and do so in a way that coincides with your activity level. The more you exercise and the more intense that exercise, the more you can get away with in your nutrition.

Many people think it's hard or it takes some secret formula. That is not the case at all. In addition, EVERYONE who has gone through one of our challenges at the gym or sat in our nutrition classes understands this fully!

As you begin this new journey in life, don't be that person sitting across from your doctor listening to how you are in the early stages of Alzheimer's, diabetes, high blood pressure/cholesterol, or, heaven forbid, a victim of cancer.

What you do today determines your health tomorrow.

The biggest misconception is people think because they "feel" okay or "look" healthy they are healthy on the inside. This is not always the case.

The same thing that causes a sliced apple to turn brown is the same thing wreaking havoc inside your own body, oxidation and inflammation. Moreover, most of these issues occur due to poor eating habits.

Imagine sitting across from your doctor after an annual physical. Picture the concerned look on his face as he tells you life is about to change forever. You can fill in the blank, but fill it with a life changing illness. It could be cancer, diabetes, heart disease, or Alzheimer's. No matter what the disease, you now find yourself a victim of what could have been a preventable. All you needed to do was make few better lifestyle choices.

In an online New York Times article titled "High Mortality from Alzheimer's Disease," in 2010 approximately 84,000 deaths were caused by Alzheimer's. They also reported close to 500,000 deaths were caused by pneumonia from complications in Alzheimer patients.

This is only one example of why prevention should be the focus. Please do not become another statistic.

Chapter 2

WHAT IS ALZHEIMER'S

There is no darkness in the presence of God's light

The following story comes from one of Poppies' daughters, Kathy. If you have been around anyone with Alzheimer's, you probably have a story that relates.

> "We were getting ready to go on a cruise to celebrate Pam and Marshall's anniversary - it's February 7, 2011. I went to mom and dad's house to bring them dinner. Dad jumps up in the middle of eating and takes me into the kitchen in the corner; he whispers "hey, what's that thing you are supposed to get your wife this week?" I look at him and say, "You mean a valentine?" He says, "Ya, get me one of those before you leave, I need one!"

Most Americans (close to 50%) believe Alzheimer's is a normal part of aging. They will end up accepting this statistic, living life as they do, in a sense waiting for the signs of dementia to appear. Walking through life with a mindset of, "If it does not affect me right now, the why worry?"

This is a dangerous attitude to have. With the increased amounts of processed foods, stress in both the home and business, and with the lack of exercise, Alzheimer's will come knocking on your door sooner than you think.

However, there are things you can do to help prevent yourself (or loved ones) from becoming another statistic of this horrible disease.

Families become divided, frustrated, at a loss of hope and loss of words when a loved one is diagnosed with Alzheimer's. Many have no idea how to cope, even when someone close to them becomes disease ridden.

Honestly, it was not until I decided to tackle the book project when dementia started to make sense. I had limited knowledge about many aspects of the disease.

Alzheimer's Appeared on the Horizon

Even a century later, Alzheimer's disease is one in its infancy stage. It did not just start to rear its ugly head; it is one of the most difficult diseases to understand. As of the spring of 2014, new research is proving a person's social environment may determine whether they develop Alzheimer's.

Later in the book, I will uncover some of the latest facts in regards to this research. In a sense, these studies can be extremely encouraging. With this type of knowledge, your chances of curing (or better put) preventing Alzheimer's will increase drastically.

One question scientists look to answer is how much of the food movement from the 80's and beyond play in the increasing development of this disease. For everything we try, there is a learning curve involved. The swing in the food movement is no different. It can take several years, if not decades, to see the ramifications of how we change the way we process food. In some cases, it could take up to a generation for side effects to become apparent.

Medications, food additives, the way food is processed, and even the way food is grown play a role in what happens to the people who consume it. Nevertheless, we will not see the ramifications of our actions unless there was a blatant disregard.

For those who suffer from Alzheimer's, the world can become a dark place. In the case of the sufferer, they may forget. For the rest of us, we may just stand there with our hands in the air asking, *"WHY?"*

None of us can comprehend the will of God as long as we walk this planet. I often ask myself why certain things happen such as handicap children, children born with cancer...etc.

Millions of people – to this day – have little knowledge of Alzheimer's. Whether it's the cause, how or who is most susceptible is all speculative. However, there are contributing factors in both speeding up the process and bettering your preventative chances.

One of the driving forces behind finding a cure is the fact that every 67 seconds someone is facing an Alzheimer's diagnosis. Alzheimer's is the most common cause of dementia and affects more than 40 million people around the world. However, finding an actual tumor is something eluding researchers today.

During the early 1900's Dr. Alois Alzheimer (a German Psychiatrist) first described symptoms after noticing a certain hospital patient had unusual problems, such as sleeping difficulties, disturbed memory, drastic mood changes and increasing confusion.

When the patient passed away, Alzheimer performed an autopsy to see if there were any irregularities in the brain's structure. Later, the symptoms Dr. Alzheimer identified as causing the eventual death of specific patients would become known as Alzheimer's disease.

During the autopsy, Dr. Alzheimer noticed dense deposits surrounding nerve cells in the brain. Inside these nerve cells, he also observed twisted bands of fibers or neurofibrillary tangles. These deposits (called neuritic plaques) occur when tangles start to develop in the brain. Eventually, these tangles begin to kill off brain cells, never to function or be replaced again.

There is often some confusion between Alzheimer's and dementia. Here is the simplest way I have heard it described.

If you look at dementia as a symptom, Alzheimer's would be the cause of that symptom. Just like an elevated body temperature is a symptom of a fever revealing some type of sickness; it does not provide any information to the cause of the sickness.

Meaning dementia is not the actual disease, but only a symptom of the disease. Everything from genetics, to lifestyle, to stress, to nutrition can come into play. Like many other diseases, there is no one factor for its cause.

Now that we understand the difference between dementia and Alzheimer's, let us look at why Alzheimer's can occur.

Misfolded Proteins & Alzheimer's

One aspect of this disease continuing to elude researchers is how the Alzheimer's process begins. Once the deadly Alzheimer's cycle begins, the damage to the brain can start at least a decade before the symptoms become apparent.

Teaching people how to take care of themselves in the present tense has been a passion of mine for some time. I have taken the approach that the earlier you address your life style choices, the better your chances at preventing life threatening disease.

The number of people who continue to live a destructive lifestyle baffles me. They tend to wave off simple lifestyle changes as if they were brushing off a fly from their shoulder. Just as with every other disease plaguing the human race, toxic changes take place inside the body long before you know you are sick.

In the case of Alzheimer's, this toxic change is taking place inside your brain. As the toxicity increases, the functions of proteins change and begin to form amyloid plaques and tau tangles. This process occurs throughout the brain as the disease spreads.

If you were to analyze these troubled proteins through a microscope, you would see they are the primary part of every living cell; otherwise known as the functional parts of cells. Over the course of a person's lifetime, some normal proteins could malfunction. Research shows this malfunction occurs due to oxidative stress. This oxidation brings on toxicity resulting in protein malfunction. This protein malfunction is called misfolding in the case of an Alzheimer patient.

Long chain amino acids make up each protein. This chain folds into a unique shape allowing interaction with other proteins and molecules. The protein APP (Amyloid Precursor Protein) is crucial in brain neuron growth and repair.

As APP's job is finished, it leaves a trail of pieces of amyloid-beta peptide. In the case of Alzheimer's, the scraps become misfolded and stick together. Eventually the scraps turn to toxic goo, resulting in large plaques.

Once these plaques take shape they start to destroy brain neurons blocking communication between cells. These once healthy neurons start to work less efficiently and stop communicating with each other all together.

As the damage spreads, the part of the brain called the hippocampus becomes affected. Once this happens you start to develop long-term memory, short-term memory, and spatial orientation problems often providing the initial Alzheimer's diagnosis.

As more neurons die, the parts of the affected areas of the brain start to shrink. Once the individual has reached the final stages the brain would have shrunk considerably. The result is complete cell death causing progressive dementia and eventually death to the individual.

Who Can Suffer From Alzheimer's?

For the last decade, Alzheimer's appeared to be a senior disease. Something most will have to deal with when they get older. However, early onset cases have appeared in individuals as early as 30 years old.

That's very different from being a senior disease!

By definition, early onset occurs before the age of 65. Most people who develop early onset (sometimes referred as younger onset) suffer from sporadic Alzheimer's disease. (I will cover the difference between sporadic and familial Alzheimer's more in-depth in Chapter 4.)

Though genetics has not proven to play a role in developing the disease, there are risk genes that increase the likelihood.

Does Alzheimer's Happen More in Men or Women

There is no question age and gender play a big factor in determining whether you develop Alzheimer's. Women have more than a 2 to 1 chance of developing Alzheimer's than men. The reason is yet to be determined.

Many theories arrived over the years and one belief was women lived longer than men did. This can be the case to an extent. There is no question the longer a person lives the better the chance of developing the disease. That can hold true for any disease.

Research has determined estrogen plays a big role in developing the disease. As women age, their physiology changes to where estrogen does not provide the protection from toxicity as it does for younger women. Many estrogenic therapies, (like Ginkgo Biloba) have proven ineffective.

Estrogen plays an important role in brain function. The brain can contain more than 100 billion neurons. Each neuron influences brain function through estrogen receptors, located on multiple areas of the brain. Estrogen can protect isolated neurons from temporary blood blockage, oxidative stress, and damage by amyloid protein. It also helps with repairing damaged neurons and growth of new neurons.

To Conclude

Science has come a long way since the discovery of Alzheimer's in the early 1900's. The human body is a remarkable specimen, but still misunderstood. What we do understand is there are specific warning signs for dementia. In order to offer you or a loved one the best chances at prevention, you have to recognize them early.

In Chapter 3, we will cover 10 warning signs.

Chapter 3

The Warning Signs

"The second half of a man's life is made up of nothing but the habits

he has acquired the first half."

> ```
> Alzheimer's impairs your ability to remember words
> when you most need them: Dad asked for, "Those
> things that you put things in that you don't want
> anymore."  He was talking about garbage bags.
> ```

There is no question the development of Alzheimer's will disrupt a person's life. It affects everyone around them. However, there are two questions people ask when the disease first appears in their life.

1. How do they function daily with the disease?

2. How do they keep from being a burden to the family as the disease progresses?

How is life affected?

Imagine waking up one day and you cannot remember where you put your car keys. On the surface, this may not seem like a big problem. However, add this to other absent-minded instances such as…

…forgetting where you were driving while you were already on your way. How about getting lost and not knowing how to get where you were going? On the other hand, how about forgetting the names of common things you use every day?

As you will learn on the next page, these are just a few of the signs to watch out for in the case of early onset Alzheimer's.

When you are in your 30's, it is easy to joke with friends, and family for that matter, but there may be a serious underlying issue at hand. Being cognizant of Alzheimer's in your family history as well as paying attention to lifestyle can reveal your chances of developing the disease.

The 10 Warning Signs of Alzheimer's

1. A Disrupted Life and Memory Loss

Ask anyone who has forgotten something and I will show you some form of memory loss. The difference between a young adult forgetting where they placed the keys is much different from say the 40, 50, 60, 70, or 80 year old who forgot something they just learned.

One of the most noticeable signs of Alzheimer's is forgetting key points of information. For instance, forgetting important dates and events; repeatedly asking for the same information; constantly needing memory aids (electronic devices or sticky notes) or needing help from family members when doing the things they use to do on their own.

For the Alzheimer's patient, older memories might seem unaffected. Recent experiences on the other hand, can be another issue. People suffering from dementia will have a problem recalling an entire event.

On the other hand, age-related memory loss may occur when trying to remember parts of an event, but later remembering them.

The Alzheimer patient will have a tendency to repeat stories no matter how many times they told it to the same person. They may also keep asking you the same questions no matter how many times answered.

With Poppie, Carole and I would joke about how he would tell me the same stories on our visits. He would tell me about his days in the Navy as a cook, then as a baker making donuts. I never grew old of the stories, but only wished I had recognized what was going on at the time.

2. Planning & Problem Solving Challenges

Another good sign Alzheimer's is setting in is when your planning and problem-solving skills deteriorate. If you are having difficulty concentrating and find yourself taking much longer to do tasks you found easy before, you may be in the initial stages of developing Alzheimer's.

For example, someone who has a hard time following a recipe or paying bills regularly can be a cause for concern. This is not to be confused with making an occasional error when balancing a checkbook. These problems can persist and become a headache for everyone involved if overlooked over time.

3. Difficulty Completing Common Tasks at Home, at Work or at Leisure

Completing daily tasks can become a nightmare for anyone on the cusp of Alzheimer's. Everything from difficulties in driving to a familiar location to managing a budget at work to remembering rules to a favorite game; these common tasks become extremely difficult.

Occasionally needing help would be more of a normal aging process.

There have been cases where people in high-level job positions get to a point where they cannot take care of their lawn – let alone continue at a job. This sign alone can be the one most frustrating to the sufferer. As a species, we do not like change. Even if that means living in denial that a problem exists.

If you find yourself fitting any of these signs, do not hesitate in getting checked.

4. Confusion: Time or Place

Another warning sign of Alzheimer's is your constantly losing track of dates, seasons and passages of time. You may have trouble understanding something you were immediately told. Forgetting where they are or how they got there are other causes of time or place confusion.

Normal aging may forget the day of the week but remember it later on.

5. Trouble with Visual Images and Spatial Relationships

For many, developing vision problems can be a natural part of aging. For the Alzheimer's patient, they have a hard time judging distance, reading, determining contrast, and colors causing problems with their driving.

One day you wake up and your eyes have a hard time functioning. You notice it takes more time to focus as you try to read what was once easy. Color, contrast, and even recognizing words can be difficult.

As the disease progresses, something as simple as looking in the mirror can become a challenge. Often they will look at their own reflection and think someone else is in the room. This same issue can transfer to mealtime as they can have a hard time distinguishing food from the plate it is placed on.

People who experience normal aging may develop vision changes. These normal changes relate more to cataracts than dementia.

6. Problems with Speaking & Writing

As writing and speaking become an issue, Alzheimer's is on the cusp of rearing its ugly head. Have you ever found yourself at a loss of words? Especially when you needed to be quiet in the past, but no one could keep you quiet. What about stopping in the middle of a sentence and had no idea how to continue the conversation. Maybe it was you repeating yourself and having trouble with finding the right word.

Struggling with the right words or calling things by their wrong names are strong indicators you may need to be evaluated for Alzheimer's. Everyone does this on occasion. Even I do this while in my 40's.

People suffering from dementia will experience severe problems remembering the most basic of words. They could become hard to follow while they speak, as it seems their speech is all over the place.

7. Misplacing objects and unable to retrace your steps

Just like in the story of my father-in-law at the beginning of this book, things that once had their place appear to have lost their place.

Better put, you can't remember where they go. If I had not watched the entire event of him putting the dishes away, I may not have believed it myself.

How many times have you misplaced your keys? Even those who are in their 20's have experienced losing something. The difference between them and developing Alzheimer's; they are not able to retrace their steps.

They may get lost in places they know. For instance, they may forget their way around their own neighborhood. They will also have problems completing basic tasks that are familiar to them – such as cooking and shaving.

In the case of misplacing objects, Alzheimer's patients will often put objects away in the wrong places. Placing a toothbrush in the fridge or a gallon of milk in a cabinet may seem normal to them.

Recently, we were reminiscing about a story after Poppie and Marge moved out of their home and into a senior care center. When the kids went back to clean out all of their personal belongings, they found silverware, bowls, cookware, etc. in the most obscure places. Marge was laughing as we told the story. She could not figure out why she was missing so many kitchen objects. Come to find out, Bob had been putting them away in the wrong places for quite some time.

8. Decreased or Poor Judgment

What was once an easy decision now seems to resemble rocket science. Giving large amounts of money to telemarketers is a prime example. Grooming and keeping themselves clean may become less of a priority as the disease progresses.

This will become obvious when someone who paid particular attention to how they looked (dressed sharply and extremely hygienic) start to wear stained clothes and may even stop bathing. However, this is not to be confused with making a bad judgment occasionally.

9. Withdrawal from social activities and work

Once someone starts to experience Alzheimer symptoms, there will be an inherent choice to remove themselves from activities they once loved. It can be anything from hobbies they once enjoyed, to avoiding social activities, work or sports events.

I can tell you this from experience as my father-in-law started to progress in his disease. He was a big Minnesota Vikings fan. Whenever we would go visit him on Sunday's he would watch the Vikings game if televised or would keep up with the score.

His interest in the Vikings slowly began to subside as he progressed deeper in his Alzheimer's. He would no longer keep up with his favorite hobbies and eventually became irritated at social events. In many cases, Alzheimer's patients are not able to understand the changes going on in their body making social settings uncomfortable.

Family members must be attuned to these changes and understand how to help the individual cope with the situation.

10. Mood & Personality Swings

One frustrating aspect of identifying Alzheimer's – especially when family and friends do not understand what is going on – is the sudden change in mood and personality.

Constant confusion, depression, suspicion, anxiousness, and being fearful are all signs the disease is taking root. They may get upset easily at home, at work, with friends or in places out of their comfort zone.

This is not to be confused with developing specific ways of doing things and becoming irritable if disrupted. That is more age-related than disease related.

People suffering from dementia may express sudden mood swings for no sensible reason. At the turn of a hat, they can become emotional, upset or angry. They become withdrawn and uncharacteristically suspicious of family members. Some even become more trusting of telemarketers, which there had been cases where their entire savings was lost because of trusting the wrong person.

For family members, it is easy to notice a change in someone's personality. They become increasingly moody, lose their temper faster than usual and tend to be more withdrawn.

Even the most introverted can become more withdrawn once Alzheimer's starts to set in. Most of the time they do not understand what is going on around them. They become fearful. They do not understand the reasoning for all the noise and commotion going on around them.

It is human nature to protect ourselves from the unknown. In addition, depending on the level of Alzheimer's depends on the level of protection they need to provide for themselves.

The key here is to try to explain what is going on. To be as comforting to them as possible; to always reassure them things are okay. The Alzheimer patient looks for familiarity, though this can be a difficult task since everything can be new to them every morning.

When to Be Evaluated

For many of us, the standard signs of Alzheimer's can be deceiving, especially if they occur sporadically. It's after each of the signs appear on a regular basis that you need to consider an evaluation by your medical professional.

Once you decide you need an evaluation, be prepared to answer the following questions when your Doctor asks them:

- What symptoms have you noticed? When did they begin?

- How often do these symptoms occur?

- Have they progressed? (Are caregivers or family members present when these symptoms occur?)

How to Be Evaluated

Instead of trying to recreate the wheel here, I have decided to give you a web link proven more beneficial than anything I can write. While searching online for answers to my own questions, I came across a great resource. This site offers five memory tests you or your loved one can take. These tests are easy to complete for those who do not suffer from any signs of Alzheimer's or dementia.

If you have problems with answering the questions correctly, it may be time to see your Doctor.

From Alzheimer's Reading Room: 5 Memory Tests. (http://www.alzheimersreadingroom.com/p/test-your-memory-for-alzheimers-5-best.html)

What to do if diagnosed

Just as with any other disease, an Alzheimer's diagnoses can initially seem like the end of the world. However, 90% of the time we, as humans, tend to blow things out of proportion in our own mind.

Making problems bigger than they are is a human trait God did not place in us. Worry is even considered a sin in the bible.

Your goal is to get over the initial shock and grieving process as quickly as possible. Remember, we are trying to protect your mind. You must get to that task as quickly as possible.

One of the many reasons why I am writing this book is to offer whatever help I can to my lovely wife Carole. Alzheimer's runs deep in her family as her dad is living in the later stages now, as well as an uncle and an aunt who died from Alzheimer's within a year of writing this book.

Prevention is the key and it starts with today!

What are the consequences to the family?

No one wants to be a burden to the people they love. Often many will hide their symptoms in order to prevent themselves from becoming that burden to the ones they care about most. This is more harmful than not; especially if you prolong getting the tests required to determine an Alzheimer's diagnoses. In the case of prevention, the earlier you can start to make lifestyle changes the better your chances of living a longer, normal life.

This brings me to the scope of this book. The more people I can get their hands on this material the better. A healthy lifestyle can be contagious. It is full of life, vigor, energy, productivity along will many other beneficial traits. Health is infectious. Just as with a virus or bacteria, you can catch health, but it has to be intentional.

You have to be an example!

Therefore, if you find yourself reading this book, and experience any of the previous mentioned warning signs, talk to your Doctor and get checked immediately. If diagnosed with early onset Alzheimer's, start to practice the lessons in Section II in this book immediately.

The section on food would be your first best bet, then exercise, lifestyle, stress, and brain stimulation. Taking Alzheimer's head on can be a daunting task. Nevertheless, if you put your mind to it, it can happen. You just have to take that first step.

Life and the consequences of bad choices

No one likes to live with the consequences of bad choices. However, bad choices only compound themselves over time with no accountability.

Your spouse and your kids may not see all the warning signs you may be hiding. In addition, because of your bad choices, there can be rough waters ahead and no one (including you) has a real understanding as to why they are happening.

Alzheimer's sufferers may not realize they are doing anything wrong at the time they are doing it. What adds to the confusion is when the consequence comes knocking at their door and no one knows the reason why.

If you find yourself in hot water because you are not sure of what you are doing, it may be time to talk to someone. You never know; it may lead to a new breakthrough or new endeavor that proves to be beneficial to everyone involved.

In chapter 4 we are going to go a little deeper into early onset Alzheimer's. The number of people who are suffering from the early stages of this disease – and have no clue they suffer from early onset Alzheimer's – is staggering.

Chapter 4

Early Onset Alzheimer's – It's NOT Just an Old Person Disease

*"I will stand by you, I will help you through when you've done all you can do, and you can't cope I will dry your eyes, I will fight your fight, I will hold you tight, and I won't let you go." – **Author unknown***

```
Dad says to me as he is talking to me on his cell
phone, "I think you have my cell, I can't find
it!"

Kathy
```

Far too many young people are noticing problems in their cognitive ability. What many do not know is there may be some cause for concern.

Instead of blowing it off as a good story for the water cooler, it should be something to pay attention to more closely if it persists. If you are one of the approximate 200,000 people diagnosed with early onset Alzheimer's, the more you know the better your chances at slowing down the disease.

As you will learn in section II, there are a number of ways where you can help prevent it (and slow down the progression) if you are suffering from the early stages of this disease.

First, let us cover some facts about who can develop Alzheimer's disease.

Genetics – What Are The Chances?

Genetic scientists have distinguished a difference between two types of Alzheimer's cases - familial and sporadic Alzheimer's.

As you can probably guess, **"Familial Alzheimer's"** is that which runs in the family - or better known as inherited through genetics. Up to 50 percent of these cases are caused by defects in three genes housed in three different chromosomes.

These structures hold the genetic code to your individual make up. In some family cases, a mutation of APP (amyloid precursor protein) causes the production of an abnormal form of the amyloid protein.

In other family cases, mutations in a gene known as presenilin 1 caused abnormal production of presenilin 1 protein. In a third type of familial Alzheimer's, scientists found a mutation in a similar gene called presenilin 2. This mutation causes the production of an abnormal presenilin 2 protein.

Okay, now that I have more than likely lost you, let me put this in more simplistic terms.

If one of these genetic mutations is present in an individual (in at least one of the two genes inherited from their parents), they will unavoidably develop that specific form of early-onset Alzheimer's.

The reassuring news is there had only been between 100 and 200 cases of this type of Alzheimer's reported worldwide. Scientists continue to work on finding out how the mutations of APP and presenilin's affect the onset of familial Alzheimer's disease. Less than 5% of cases are true familial Alzheimer's disease.

Sporadic Alzheimer's on the other hand is a more common type of the disease. Again, genetics does appear to play a role in this type of Alzheimer's. In this version, the gene at hand is called APOE (apolipoprotein E). There are different variations of these genes that produce bodily characteristics such as blood type and eye color.

What researchers realized is they needed to pay attention to the variations in the APOE gene. One of the functions of this gene is to direct the manufactured apolipoprotein E to carry blood cholesterol throughout the body.

In a healthy brain, APOE is in your neurons and other supportive brain cells (called glia). However, in excess amounts it is associated with the plaques found in the brains of people with Alzheimer's.

As of late, researchers are starting to pay particular attention to three common alternative forms of the APOE gene: e2, e3, and e4. In regards to the discovery of the APOE e4 gene, it has helped explain several variations in the age of onset Alzheimer's.

This due to whether the individual has inherited none...one...or two copies of the APOE e4 allele from their parents. The more APOE e4 alleles a person inherits, the younger the disease onslaught.

As to APOE e2 allele - though relatively rare – it has shown to protect some against the disease. There seems to be a lower risk connected to developing young onset Alzheimer's as well as developing it at a later age.

The APOE e3 is found in the general population and appears to play a neutral role in Alzheimer's.

So, who carries the APOE gene that develops Alzheimer's disease?

One thing is for sure, there is no certainty to who develops it, or if they do. Some people can carry APOE e4 alleles and avoid ever having any signs of dementia. It does increase the chances of developing the disease, but does not cause it. Scientists continue to research how genetics contributes (or does not) to an individual developing any form of dementia.

Several theories exist, including interactions with cholesterol levels and effects on nerve cell death. Only time will tell as research continues.

What Would You Do?

Think about this for a minute. Imagine you are a high-level executive working at the "C" level in a fortune 500 company. Your day normally consisted of you driving to work, drinking your coffee and answering text messages as you head into the office. (Of course, I do not encourage you to try this at home.)

You are a 40 year old male and at the top of your game. However, you have been noticing changes in your ability to perform what you consider the mundane tasks.

Tasks like remembering phone conversations, remembering where your office was located and remembering to make an employee meeting you arranged.

This is only one of the countless examples taken from a PBS special titled "Suffers of Early Onset Alzheimer's Describe Life with the Disease." If you have any thought something is off with your cognitive abilities, I encourage you to follow the link and read some of the stories.

I cannot help but think this problem will be of pandemic proportions as the after effects of the Fat-free era of the 1980's starts to set in. Researchers continue to show the importance food plays in our overall health. Only time will tell as the aftermath of that era begins to play out its role in our society.

Chemicals, overly processed foods, processing techniques themselves, all play a role in the toxicity of our overall health. I have no problem stating eventually science will determine everything from cosmetics, to air pollution, to food, and lifestyle will determine our mental state in our later years.

If you are in your thirties and have some concern then take control of your health IMMEDIATELY! My biggest concern is the people who need to see this type of resource will not see it - eventually becoming another statistic.

Rates of Progression

Each case of Alzheimer's is unique. People who tend to be unsocial, unable to handle stress effectively, eat poorly, lives a sedentary life, suffer from other diseases - as well as other life-style traits - can experience faster growth of Alzheimer's. Those with the disease, on average, live eight years, though some have lived with the disease for twenty years. One crucial key is how early you are diagnosed, and if steps are taken to slow down the progression.

Here is a generalized breakdown of Alzheimer's*:*

Early onset Alzheimer's - changes could occur in their 30's...40's...50's...etc. before diagnosis.

Mild to moderate Alzheimer's - will typically last 2 - 10 years.

Severe Alzheimer's - could last 1 - 5 years.

High Cholesterol

You've heard it before, keep your cholesterol level in check or pay the consequences down the road. Diet, weight, physical activity, and exposure to tobacco smoke can affect your cholesterol level.

High Blood Pressure

Research is showing high blood pressure can play an intricate role in developing Alzheimer's. More specifically, vascular dementia (a common form of dementia caused by an impaired supply of blood to the brain may be caused by a series of small strokes) appears to be increased as heart or blood vessels are damaged.

Symptoms such as high blood pressure, heart disease, stroke, diabetes, and high cholesterol can affect your heart brain connection. Any impairment in the amount of blood flow making its way to your brain increases your chances of dementia.

These same studies show that the tangles and plaques are more likely to cause Alzheimer's symptoms if strokes or damage to the brain's blood vessels are also present.

To Conclude

In this chapter, I covered how genes can play an intricate role in development of Alzheimer's. Over the course of one's life, there are contributing factors that either increase or decrease your chances. In the case of early onset, the earlier you recognize, act upon, and change your key life-style habits, the better chances of protecting your mind down the road.

I know I may sound like a broken record, but I cannot emphasize the importance of you taking a proactive approach to your health, now.

In chapter 5, I will go into head injuries and what role they play in dementia.

Chapter 5

It's All In Your Head

Indeed, you are my lamp, O Lord, the Lord lightens my darkness. --2 Samuel 22:29

Soon after, mom said the nursing home put a doorbell on their door. Every time someone would enter or exit the doorbell would ring. They figured this would work so they wouldn't lose dad again.

Well dad being the ornery boy that he is thought it was really funny to sit at the door and move his walker back and forth across the floor so that the doorbell rang constantly!

Carole

Can head injuries expedite Alzheimer's?

There seems to be a direct correlation between traumatic head injuries and the development of Alzheimer's (and dementia) later in life. Effects of a head injury could include; confusion, unconsciousness, inability to remember the traumatic event, trouble speaking (mumbling), unsteadiness, trouble remembering new information, trouble with coordination, hearing, and vision problems.

Older adults who have had repeated moderate head injuries are twice as likely to be at risk of developing Alzheimer's disease. Those with a history of traumatic head injuries have four times a greater chance of developing the disease.

Evidence is suggesting that repeated mild traumatic head injuries from sports such as; football, hockey, soccer, and boxing may increase the chance of a type of dementia called chronic traumatic encephalopathy.

Traumatic head injuries change the brain's chemistry. Everything from vehicle crashes, falls (where your head hits an object or ground), and sports injuries are showing to increase dementia and Alzheimer's cases. The better you can protect yourself the better your chances of avoiding an increased risk of suffering from these diseases.

Can you recover from a head injury?

The adult human brain weighs about 3 pounds and is made of extremely soft tissue. The makeup of your brain allows it to be pulled, squeezed (compressed), and stretched. This soft tissue sits inside your skull and floats in a protective fluid. Inside the skull resides three layers of membrane covering and protecting the brain.

As you experience a traumatic event such as a car crash, sports injury, or fall, there is a sudden speeding up and slowing down of the head's movement. Your brain can move violently inside your skull causing traumatic damage.

Your recovery from such a traumatic event will depend on the extent of the injury (or its repetitiveness).

This results in changes in thinking and behavior. It can take weeks and sometimes months for the brain to resolve the chemical imbalance that occurs with a traumatic brain injury. As the brain's chemistry improves, so can the person's ability to function properly. This is one reason that someone may make rapid progress in the first few weeks after an injury.

To say our brains are delicate would be an understatement. Neurotransmitters (chemical substances in the brain) must be able to communicate with certain cells in the central nervous system. During normal functions, chemical signals are sent from neuron-to-neuron. Groups of these neurons work with each other to perform normal functions.

A brain injury disrupts this delicate chemistry preventing the neurons from working normally. This changes your thinking and behavior which can take weeks (if not months) to recover from. During this recovery time, processing information will become much slower and frustrating for the individual.

Your best defense is to limit the chances of experiencing a traumatic head injury. Though there is no way to protect yourself one hundred percent, you can increase your protection level in your activities by wearing the proper safety equipment.

In Conclusion

As I mentioned earlier, Section I was to give you an overview of the disease and some of the things leading into Alzheimer's. Section II is about techniques you can apply right now to help better your chances at prevention.

Though there is no guarantee that protects you 100%, there are things you can do to help prevent you from developing the disease. If you are facing an early onset diagnosis, there are ways of slowing down the progress.

There is one thing I ask of you as you go through Section II – simply APPLY what you read. An extremely frustrating aspect of being a Fitness Professional is the fact many do not follow through; even a half-hearted approach will prove beneficial to you and your loved ones.

As you tackle Section II, start with nutrition. Then work on exercising while adding the brain games to your daily activities.

Once you begin to develop - and work - on your own 3 Pillared approach (Nutrition, Activity, and Brain Stimulation), you will notice your quality of life improve drastically.

Section II

It's Your Life Take Control of It

In section II I plan to give you a 3 Pillared Approach to helping you prevent Alzheimer's. Though each of the three pillars themselves is detrimental to your living a healthy life, it's not until you put all three in place do you optimize your chances of being disease free. (And this extends past dementias. You could rid yourself of many of the ailments you are suffering from.)

If you take and apply everything you learn here, you will help ensure you are around to enjoy your children and even grandchildren.

All I can encourage you to do is...

TAKE ACTION.

Chapter 6

The Power of Exercise

"When one door closes another door opens, but sometimes it's hell in

the hallway!"

> *Dad called and he was hollering really loud on the phone. He was trying to tell me he was having trouble changing the TV channel. I am hollering back saying I can hardly hear him. I finally say, "Dad do you have the remote on your ear and the phone for your remote?" Dad, "awe, hell ya I do..."*
>
> **Kathy**

Aaah...exercise! Either you love it or you hate it, not a whole lot in between. Exercise has been a part of my family as far back as I can remember. Growing up my parents were always involved with martial arts. Mom also taught aerobic classes a few times a week and my dad and I would spend hours on the weekends playing basketball together in the back yard.

I had no idea how to sit around and do nothing.

Every generation has their secret sauce for keeping in shape. Today it seems like anyone who can afford to pay for an infomercial spot has the new life-changing program; the end-all-be-all of fitness gimmicks.

What I am about to share with you here has come from what I have learned to call the minimalist approach.

Due to some unforeseen event that has caused scoliosis to set into my spine (along with moderate degeneration in my neck), I have been forced to look at exercise through a completely new set of eyes.

Everything I do stems around my own body weight. There is no doubt God works in His own way. Often times I can't help but believe He has put me here to better help you. Not with some crazy drawn out exercise program, but by seeing through the lines and giving you the easiest approaches to help ensure you get started.

Without further ado, let us dive into some simple life-style changes you can start today.

Can exercise reduce your risk of Alzheimer's?

The name of the game here with exercise is improving oxygen consumption. Aerobic activity (meaning you are able to hold a conversation as you workout) increases blood flow throughout the body. It benefits brain function and has shown to reduce brain cell loss in the elderly.

Some researcher's state exercise can decrease your chances of developing Alzheimer's by as much as 50%. Whether that is proven or not is yet to be seen. However, I would rather take my chances on exercising than not.

What if I've been inactive for a while – is it too late?

"It's better late than never." I have no idea as to who first made that statement, but it is one to live the test of time. I read a quote online recently that stated, *"There is plenty of time to lounge around when you are dead."*

Harsh - yes, but true.

If you find yourself feeling like you had better start exercising, take heed to what you're being told. Do not think that for a moment exercise will be easy; especially if you find yourself coming from the couch to the gym. For this new habit to stick there has to be a less painful route. Otherwise, you will find every excuse to talk yourself out of exercise.

I know this because I have done this same thing in the past.

The key is taking the time and writing down what you like to do or what you <u>would</u> do. You can walk, swim, bike, run, row, do jumping jacks, chase chickens around your yard (though your neighbors may look at you funny) or climb several flights of stairs. The key is to find something you can do and stick with it – three to five times a week.

Many experts will tell you it will take at least 21 days to establish a new habit. That is too far-sighted for me. You want to focus on right now; what you will do right now to develop new habits.

I have a saying in the gym; *"Only focus on the next rep; not the rest of the workout."*

Meaning if you focus on what you are doing today, tomorrow will take care of itself. So grab a piece of paper, a pen and write down what types of activities you would actually do. It can be a trip to the gym or a trip to a school to play soccer or basketball, the key is doing something.

What are the benefits to exercise?

Out of all the questions someone could ask on this topic, this is the easiest to answer. Exercise reduces stress, boosts mood, improves memory and increases your energy.

Can you think of anything better than taking your stress and frustrations out during your workout? Of course, this does not mean breaking gym equipment, but redirecting your stress to stop your mental downward spiral.

Stress is a nasty trait we have to deal with. Some are wired so tight just about anything can set them off. Not only does this prove hurtful to your mind, but it brings a host of other health issues.

When people come to me frustrated, tired, fed up and ready to bite the world's head off, I would tell them to leave their problems right here on the gym floor. Sounds corny I know. However, I cannot count the number of times someone told me, *"Thank you!"* after encouraging them to do this very thing.

Time after time they would literally put so much effort into their workouts they felt one hundred percent better – and left the gym with a clear head.

Imagine skipping your workout and heading straight home instead, or worse yet, to a bar. Once you got home there is a pretty good chance you would take out your frustrations on your family. In doing so, you will start to affect your most important social environment - home.

The next time you need to take out some frustration, take it out on your workout by working so hard you cannot help but feel better once you are done.

How to Get Started

The quote at the beginning of this chapter sums it up pretty well, *"When one door closes another door opens, but sometimes it's hell in the hallway!"*

The first step is always the hardest, no matter what it is in life. People will experience paralysis by analysis; there is so much information available today only confusing many.

The key to getting started is – JUST START!

Remember the list you made earlier? Go back to it and pick an activity you can do right now this very minute, even if it means putting this book down. Go do something for the next 30-45 minutes right now. This book will always be here, but there is no guarantee your health will be.

The key is blocking out 30 minutes of exercise 5 times a week. No questions, no excuses, just do it. You will begin to reap the rewards almost immediately once you start this habit.

Boost Brain Power with Balance and Coordination

Include balance and coordination in your exercise program. Having good balance and coordination is imperative to your health. When you participate in activities requiring a strict focus on balance and coordination, you force your brain to communicate with your musculoskeletal system. Your brain then is actively working every second to keep your body upright for as long as it is being challenged.

This will prove beneficial later in life as you become more susceptible to falling. As you've learned earlier in this book, it only takes one traumatic head injury to significantly increase your chances of Alzheimer's.

Simple exercises like hopscotch, heel-to-toe exercises, balancing on one leg, and even jumping rope will increase your balance and coordination capacity.

Stick with it - Believe it or not, this can be the hardest of all the habits you'll create when you follow this book. Over the years I've seen a majority of people lack the discipline to "stick with it" for the duration.

It is easy to see some results, then walk away thinking you've done everything you could do. I cannot emphasize enough the fact this will be a life-long journey.

Yes, we all fall off the bandwagon once in a while. But it is imperative we get back on as soon as possible.

If you feel inclined to blow off the rest of your life, realize this one thing...you can only get diagnosed once. Currently, once you are diagnosed, you are stuck with that diagnose the rest of your life.

It all comes down to making choices. You will not escape that. Either choose to do something, or choose to do nothing.

Make the right choice.

Exercise Examples

Before you start any exercise program make sure your Doctor approves of what you are doing. In the end, your Doctor will know your limitations. If you have underlying issues preventing you from performing certain exercise, understand there are modifications for everything.

With that, let's get to work!

Remember when you were a kid and all you would do is look for things to climb on? Trees, monkey bars, the side of garages (don't ask), etc. were all free game to play on. At some point as we got older, we lost our childlike drive to climb and play on whatever we could find.

I have some good news; to set you free…to give you permission to go to your local park and start climbing again.

Often I will drive by a park and look at their play sets. I will check out everything I can use for a workout. The beauty of this is you do not have to go to a gym. Most of you have your own play sets where your children (and grandchildren) play – right there in your own back yard.

Just get creative! Spend 20 minutes moving your own body weight around with different exercises. I will make it easy by giving you three exercises you can start doing right this very minute.

Best Body Weight Exercises

The Push-up - There is a specific reason why every branch of the military makes you do push-ups until you basically collapse flat on your face.

It is arguably the best upper body exercises for building strength, endurance and lean muscle. The push-up easily translates to everyday life. This movement requires you to work the "pushing" muscles; chest, triceps, shoulders and your core.

At last count I came up with close to 60 different push-up variations. For now, let me cover a few fundamentals for three variations of the push-up. I will cover the simplest version for the beginner first, and then moving to intermediate and finishing with advanced.

Beginner: Wall Push-up – This version is for the person new to exercise or someone with an upper body injury.

- Stand as far away from the wall as your strength allows.

- Place your hands out in front of you at chest height.

- Then slowly fall forward until your hands are firmly on the wall.

- Lower yourself towards the wall by bending at your elbows only.

- Once your face gets close to the wall, push as hard as you can until your arms are locked out again.

- Do this for as many reps as you can.

Intermediate: Knee push-up – This version is a little more advanced and can be modified a number of ways. The key here is keeping your body as flat (parallel) with the floor as possible.

- With your knees on the floor (or on a pad if you have tender knees) walk your hands out until your upper body is in a straight line. Your chest, shoulder and tricep strength will determine how straight your upper body will be. Maintaining this position through the entire range of motion is your goal.

- With your head raised slightly, bend at your elbows and slowly lower your body until your chest and chin are touching the ground.

- Next, with as much force as you can, press through the palms of your hands as you press yourself up to the starting position.

- Do this for 2-3 sets of 5-10 reps starting out.

Advanced: Military push-up – Over the course of my 44 years I've done thousands of military push-ups. It's not uncommon for me to do 200-300 of these in a workout. The key here is keeping your body as straight and rigid as possible through the entire range of motion.

- With your toes on the floor walk your hands out until your entire body is in a straight line.

- With your head raised slightly begin the movement by bending your elbows. Continue this downward motion until your chest and chin are touching the ground.

- Next, with as much force as you can, press through the palms of your hands as you push yourself up to the starting position.

- Once you are at this level you can perform at least 3-5 sets of as many reps as you can without stopping.

As long as you maintain safe form, you can let your imagination run when it comes to push-ups. You can add resistance by wearing a weighted vest; increase the angle by doing handstand push-ups or do as many as you can in two minutes.

Push-ups can be done every day if you choose to do them.

The Squat – This basic movement gets overlooked due to its simplicity. I am mesmerized by the number of people who view the squat as an exercise and not an activity done several times a day.

For instance, getting in and out of a chair is nothing more than a squat. How many times do you go to the bathroom a day? Guess what? You squatted!

The key to this fundamental movement is to protect your knees. What many call a squat are really only partial squats that place too much pressure on the knee joint. The next time you sit down and get up from a chair, remember these tips to a perfect squat.

- Stand with your feet about shoulder width apart.

- Make sure your toes are angled out slightly. If you were to draw a straight line through each foot (running from beyond your toes to beyond your heal), as you looked down you would see the letter "V."

- As you start to sit back (squat) move your hips back first. Imagine you are sitting down in a chair. Continue to move your hips back and down to where your rear end is below your knees.

- While keeping your head tall, chests tall, and your weight on your heels, press yourself up to the standing position by placing all your weight on the heels of your feet.

Here is one of the easiest ways to get a squat workout in at least three days a week.

During your favorite 30-minute television show, practice these squatting techniques during each of the 2-3 commercial breaks. Once you get comfortable with the movement, you can try to better your reps each attempt. You can make it a game by trying to beat your previous attempt.

Toe Touches – Most people hate stretching and will avoid it like the plague. What many fail to realize is several injuries will stem from tight muscles.

I know this may seem a little far-fetched, but hear me out.

Talk to most chiropractors and they can tell you a lot of your back issues can originate from tight hamstrings and a weak core.

Humans were created to move. For our hunter and gatherer ancestors, movement was crucial to survival. I'm sure they had back problems on occasion; not because they sat at a desk for hours on end. Can you imagine trying to lift (and move) a large kill all by yourself? I am sure Gog may have jacked up his back a time or two in those days.

Over time our body starts to tighten up as it becomes less active. Hips, torso, hamstrings and back all work together in unison in order to move. Once movement stops, each of these areas will tense (or tighten) causing strain on the neighboring areas.

Meaning, as your hamstrings tighten, your pelvis is pulled down and away from your lumbar spine. This in turn puts your lower back in an unstable position. Your goal is to prevent this from occurring – or to reverse this issue if it has started.

The key to stretching your hamstrings is to keep your legs as straight as possible through the entire range of motion. The straighter the leg the deeper the hamstring stretch.

You can perform toe touches from the standing position, seated position or lying on your back.

- From the standing position bring your feet together.
- Keep your legs as straight as you can without locking the knees.
- Slowly lower your body (walking your hands down the front of the body) as far as you can. Once you feel a slight pull on the back of your thighs, hold that position for about 18-20 seconds
- Slowly stand back up

The key to this stretch is keeping your legs straight. The same teaching points apply for all three variations (standing, seated and lying on your back). Make sure you do not bounce and maintain deep, controlled breathes throughout the entire stretch.

In Conclusion

Each of these three simple exercises can be done anywhere. Whether in your living room, the park, the gym, you name it; you can get a great workout in faster than you ever imagined.

Now keep in mind this is only three of thousands of different exercises. I could easily make this another exercise book, but who really needs that?

Remember; just get started by taking some type of action right now.

Bonus Section - Sleep

Recovery is just as important as the time you spend working out. For all the years I've been in and out of gyms, people seem to have the same misconceptions; you build lean muscle when you work out in the gym and the longer the workouts the better.

WRONG! The exact opposite holds true.

For optimum health, you need to rest much more than you workout. Your body builds lean muscle mass during your rest periods (outside of the gym). While in the gym, you are breaking down muscle tissue. It is at rest when the body repairs itself. Getting 7-8 hours of quality sleep every night will help ensure your body will recover fully from the previous days stress.

Relaxation techniques to help you get a good night's rest – Though what you are about to read may seem far-fetched, they work well in helping you get that much needed rest. The best way to make them work is to follow each exercise to its completion.

You will know these techniques worked the next morning after waking from a peaceful night's rest.

Body Tensing – On the surface this could appear to have the opposite effect. The best way to relax your body is after it has been tense. As you release tension, focus on relaxing the area previously tensed. You will have better body awareness, which helps you to relax at a deeper level.

- While lying on your back – you can start anywhere on the body – pick a group of muscles and squeeze them. Hold for a 2-3 second count, and then totally relax.

- Do this same thing with another group of muscles and continue until you drift off into la-la-land.

Body Relaxation – This is very similar to the body tensing technique with one major difference. Here you want to totally relax every muscle in the body without tensing. This will put your mind and body at ease and allow you to fall into a nice deep sleep.

- While on your back place your hands down to your sides.

- Starting with your toes, totally relax them and only them.

- Then move to your entire foot. As you are starting to relax, imagine you are melting into your mattress. Almost like you are sinking in quicksand.

- As your feet relax, move up each leg and continue to do the same thing until you feel your entire body sinking into the mattress.

I've practiced this specific technique when my head is racing keeping me up all night. I normally fall asleep before I get to my thighs.

Counting backwards - This is a new spin on counting sheep. This one takes some concentration. It helps prevent you from thinking of other things while you lay there in bed staring at the ceiling. Eventually you get in a rhythm and usually fall asleep before hitting the end of the countdown.

- This is very simple, start counting backwards by 3's – starting at 300. Example: 300…297…294…291…etc.

So much of our lives become a mental game. We play these games with ourselves all the time. However, knowing when to recognize them, and what to do about them makes life much easier. Try any one of these techniques and note how well you slept through the night.

In Chapter seven, let's talk about food.

Chapter 7

Food: Your God Created Medication

"One cannot think well, love well, sleep well, if one has not dined well."

— *Virginia Woolf*

```
I went shopping for Emma's 1st birthday gift.  I
bought 4 outfits and took them to show mom and dad
to see if mom liked them.  As I'm putting each
outfit in moms lap dad is just watching and
watching.

After I was done and they said they liked them I
went to the bedroom to look for wrapping paper.  I
overheard dad say to mom, "she needs to know those
aren't going to fit you!"
```

Just as with religion, wars are started because of conflicting beliefs on food. Honestly, there is no real secret to health. Just as with exercise, everyone has the secret to last a lifetime – or at least until the next spin-off secret is created.

In some business circles they call that "modeling."

Back on point…

While I sit here to write this book, I find myself biting my own tongue. The topic of food can seriously open a nasty can of worms. However, what you will find here - in this book - is what I personally focus on. It is the same way I coach everyone I work with on the topic of nutrition.

As long as you keep it simple, follow a few simple guidelines, and stay persistent, food can literally reverse disease.

The Hunter & Gather Mentality

A Glance at the Life of Gog

Gog stood up, grabbed his spear and walked towards the entrance of his cave. While at the opening, he surveyed the horizon in front of him. With spear in hand, the sun was rising just off to the left of the cave's entrance. His family fast asleep; warm and safe. Gog knows it's time to go find today's "catch."

"I love the thrill of the hunt! Just as much as I love the smile on my family's faces as they enjoy the meal-of-the-day."

Like a man on a mission, he's off...sprinting down the hill front. His family lay nestled safely in their cave. Several thoughts run through his head, mainly the pressures of success. The previous couple of days were sparse. It's been slim-pickens with the wild game on the move for some reason.

He slows to a slow jog, needing to conserve energy. He has to be ready to strike as that ever elusive prize winning catch presents itself. The last few days have been nightmarish. His aches, his pains, amplified due to the changes in his eating.

He's tired. Hunting is hard work. His body is unable to recover without proper nourishment. The lack of protein prevents his body from repairing itself as it should.

A guy can only live on nuts and berries for so long! he thinks to himself. *But wait...there in the distance...what is that? Aaah, lunch.*

Don't get too caught up in the particulars of Gog's tale. It's only an example; a mere glimpse into our ancestry. Many would argue whether cavemen existed. Even if specific foods were around during their time in history

Imagine what life would be like if Gog had the benefits of a drive-thru. Can you imagine him riding the back of the family mammoth –

with family in tow? Slowly approaching the order speaker and placing his order…

"I'll take two # 2's, one #3 and a baby Gog # 7…all with diet sodas please."

I'm sure our existence would have ended long before we made it this far if Gog had the convenience of a drive-thru.

The more I researched Alzheimer's, the more I see how toxicity plays a tremendous role in our ultimate demise. We are exposed to more toxins through our food, our cosmetics and air pollution now than ever before – combined.

Let's briefly talk about hormones and how they play an integral part in your overall health.

The Hormone Insulin

It seems everyone is familiar with this hormone. Whether you like it or not insulin gets a negative rap. It is considered a storage hormone produced by the pancreas and is triggered by carbohydrates.

In this carb-laden society we live in, carbohydrates seem to be the staple in the standard American diet. I will give credit where credit is due; a small part of the population is paying attention to the number (and the types) of carbohydrates they eat.

Not all carbohydrates are created equal.

In order for you to keep your blood sugar at an even level throughout the day, you must regulate the amount of carbohydrates you consume. I refrain from getting into the glycemic index here, but you want the slowest digested carbohydrates you can find.

If you look at your body as a giant food processor, you can understand the denser the food, the more difficult it is to break down. The body has to work harder to break down some foods than it does others.

A simple carbohydrate is one that is easier to break down; the harder the breakdown the more complex the carbohydrate. Complex carbohydrates provide stable blood sugar level because it gets into the blood stream at a much slower pace than their simple cousins.

The best rule of thumb is to limit your carbohydrate intake to vegetables and fruit - the more local and organic the better the quality of food.

When shopping, keep to the outside perimeter of the grocery store. There you will find the best choices of vegetables and fruits, which will provide you with the much needed antioxidants to help prevent toxicity.

The Hormone Leptin

What in the world is Leptin? *(Pronounced lept-in.)*

First off let's go over the fact that both leptin and insulin work together.

Though we do not hear much about leptin in the media, it's considered a "master control" hormone and is more important than insulin.

Leptin's main job is to ensure we use enough energy and fat reserves to get us through the day. It functions to turn off appetite while promoting the burning of triglycerides that bloat fat cells. As you accumulate fat cells, leptin is bound in the blood preventing it from being transported across the blood-brain-barrier.

Basically, your brain never gets the signal to stop eating. The brain does not get the signal to burn fat storage so more fat gets accumulated. The problem only gets worse over time as we age unless we get our eating habits under control.

We use this hormone to survive famines and emergencies.

Let's go a little more in-depth about this hormone leptin:

- Leptin controls the rate of your metabolism.

- It controls how much energy you use. The more energy you have the more energy you have for other hormone production. It allows you to get into a "Thriving" state where your body is able to handle just about anything thrown at it.

- Leptin is in fat cells and is a "Fuel Gauge" for the brain.

- It tells you how much energy you have and need to use.

- It lets you know when you need more food and when you had enough.

Leptin controls the message line from your brain to your stomach. When you become leptin resistant, the cell receptors stop communicating with the cells. This in turn forces a breakdown in communication throughout the body.

Leptin resistant people will have a higher tendency to overeat as the message of feeling full never makes it to the correct "call" center.

Reversing leptin resistance is the same as reversing the other hormone issues spoken on in this book. Granted, there are always circumstances that fall out of the norm and special cases will exist. Make sure you consult a physician if there is ever a question about your health.

Now we'll wrap hormones up with the *Good Guy* hormone glucagon…

The Hormone Glucagon

We now know insulin in considered a storage hormone produced by the pancreas. In a nutshell it allows stuff into your cells. Whether it's the good (nutrients) or the bad, it's getting stuff inside the cells. It is produced in response to raised blood sugar (glucose) levels. Or simply put, carbohydrate intake.

You may be wondering, "What is glucagon's job?"

Answer: To regulate the metabolism of glucose (blood sugar) and other nutrients taken in by food.

When you go long periods of time without food, you develop what is often referred to as hunger pangs. Nine out of ten times (for the untrained person) this leads you to looking for some type of carbohydrate - and not the good kind.

When you eat those carbohydrates, they are converted to sugars in the blood. This causes the release of insulin in the blood stream.

What happens next is absolutely amazing!!

Insulin allows sugars to leave the blood and enter the cells of the body (unless the lock and key mechanism stops working due to insulin resistance.)

From there a change in your brain chemistry generates a feeling of being satisfied. Over the course of time (typically a couple hours), the insulin-to-blood sugar ratio will change yet again. This time the brain will again cause a sensation of hunger.

Let's take a look at an apple for example.

When you eat an apple, after it's digested, it will pass through your digestive system and then into your blood. It is then called blood glucose (sugar.)

Your body will then sense the sudden increase in blood glucose. From there it will signal your pancreas to release insulin. This allows, as well as helps, carbohydrates, proteins and fats to enter cells.

Now you can begin to understand why insulin is considered a storage hormone. It allows the nutrients from the blood to be stored into the cells for proper function.

This is important because each of the cell membranes (the outer parts of the cell) are made up of a couple layers of fat.

Along these membranes are receptors. These are the small door-like entrances into the cells. Through these *doors* the insulin (which can be likened to a key) unlocks the doors (which are receptors). If everything is working properly, the nutrients from your food are let into the cells via the receptors and your body will function correctly.

On the opposite side of the spectrum, we have **"Glucagon"**. And this hormone is considered a *release hormone*.

As insulin allows stuff into the cells, glucagon (the good guy hormone) allows that same stuff out of the cells. Since insulin is triggered by carbohydrates, glucagon is triggered by protein.

The real kicker here is neither can be produced in great quantities at the same time. Meaning, if there are high amounts of insulin in the blood stream then you will have low amounts of glucagon. The same can be said about large amounts of glucagon.

High insulin = low glucagon (bad)

Low insulin = high glucagon (good)

Wrapping up hormones

As you strive to create more balanced nutritional habits, make sure you focus on eating protein at every meal. This prevents your blood sugar levels from looking like your favorite roller-coaster ride.

Every time your blood sugar elevates you are in fat storage mode. For the less active person this allows body fat to accumulate over time. Much like Alzheimer's itself; this is a slow process and happens very subtly. Due to insulin's storing nature, it will allow any toxins into the cells as well. Eventually resulting in cell death, which will lead to excess inflammation…

…with the end result leading to disease.

Hydration and Alzheimer's

One question I often hear is, *"What's the big deal with water?"*

More than 50% of the entire body is made up of water. One key role is it keeps tissues, cells, and organs functioning properly as it helps transport nutrients throughout the body.

Hundreds of emergency room visits are made each year because someone is experiencing dehydration, and showing signs of dementia.

Some symptoms of dehydration can be: dry mouth, dizziness, feeling tired, rapid breathing, forgetting things, low urine output, dark yellow urine, lethargy, constipation, muscle weakness, headache, fatigue and confusion. In this case, an E.R. physician will simply prescribe liquids to help alleviate the problems.

Alzheimer's patients can experience these same types of symptoms, but due to other issues at hand. Many Alzheimer patients simply forget to drink, or they may have a swollen throat. In either case, they may not be sure how to communicate the problem with their caregiver. In the case of incontinence, they may not drink water because they do not want to go to the bathroom.

All of which will lead to dehydration of the patient.

How much do you need? The answer to this question is about as broad as any question can be. Each individual has a unique need of hydration. For seniors, at least 7 cups of water a day is enough to keep them hydrated.

For the younger population who are much more active, it can be tricky in determining how much to drink each day. One rule of thumb I like to use is simple:

Take your body weight (whatever your scale says) and divide that number by 2. The answer will give you a good starting point of how much water is enough. In the case of a 200 pound person, 100 ounces of water is a good goal to strive for each day.

How to ensure you get enough water? One of the best practices I have used here is keeping a container large enough to hold my daily requirements of water. My goal is to drink the entire container before the end of the day. I am not always successful; however it does keep me accountable.

This brings us to the end of the nutrition talk. Let us talk about something appearing to be God's new wonder drug…

Coconut Oil & Other Important Nutrients

If you were to do an internet search on dementia and coconut oil, you would be flooded with pages of people talking about the topic. In some circles coconut oil is banished because it is high in saturated fat. Research is clearly showing that it is not the saturated fat causing the health issues of today. It is the inflammation stemming from toxicity along with hormone imbalances.

Our family has used coconut oil (in large quantities) for the last few years. We use it to cook, Carole my wife, uses coconut cream in her coffee in place of a dairy creamer. We even use coconut manna (coconut butter) on sweet potatoes.

What you will learn here are the benefits of coconut oil pertaining to Alzheimer's. There is not the time or space here to cover all of the benefits of this amazingly beneficial food. But I will touch the surface.

Why Coconut Oil

Coconut oil is loaded with medium chain triglycerides from which your body makes what is known as ketones. These ketones are helpful as backup fuel for brain cells. Clinical trials are indicating these ketones can help compensate for dementia. Of course, every case is unique due to specifics of their case and the stage of dementia. For many it only takes a few weeks to see if coconut oil will help.

Quality is the key when it comes to coconut oil. There are dozens of brands aiming to provide a coconut free tasting product. You want to use the purest, organic, virgin coconut oil you can find. The taste is a by-product of the benefits. Over time you do not notice the added flavor.

How to start using Coconut Oil

Start small by mixing one teaspoon into each meal and increase the amount slowly. The best dosage seems to be working towards three tablespoons per meal and two before going to bed. Once distributed throughout the day in this matter, the peak effects are noticed within 2 hours after eating. If you experience an upset stomach, decrease the amount until the issue goes away.

Coconut oil is great when used in recipes, frying eggs, fish, and making other dishes. One thing to consider is coconut oil lacks the brain-healthy omega 3. Taking a fish oil supplement and/or eating more tuna salmon, trout and sardines will help fill that void.

In Conclusion

The name of the game with nutrition is balance. Getting enough protein, complex carbs from vegetables & fruit, and fat from healthy sources such as olive & coconut oil, fatty fish, avocados, black olives, nuts, and seeds are crucial to brain health.

Cut out as much packaged food as you can and shop at your local Farmer's Markets. There you will have the best chances of finding free-range and grass fed meats along with organic produce. A little bit can go a long way.

The Coconut Oil Clock Test

If you search coconut oil clock test online you will find some amazing research on the power of coconut oil for Alzheimer patients. The picture below shows a case where there was a significant improvement once coconut oil was introduced to the patient's nutrition.

Keep in mind every case in unique and there is no guarantee everyone will see this type of improvement. However, if you do not have any allergy issues with coconut oil, then it is worth a try.

Improvement is much better than decline!

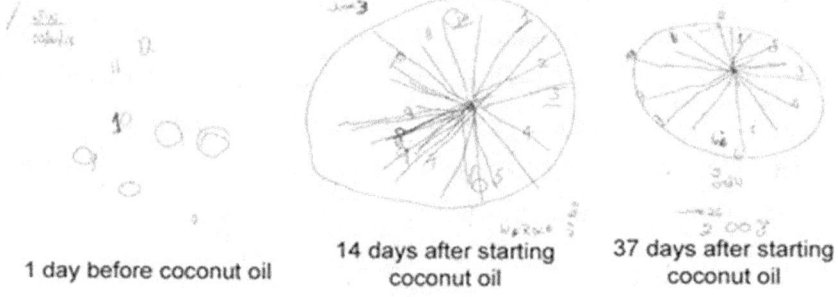

1 day before coconut oil   14 days after starting coconut oil   37 days after starting coconut oil

In the next chapter I will get a little deeper inside your brain.

Chapter 8

The Brain – Everyone's Personal Computer

*Because of the tender mercy of our God, With which the Sunrise from on high will visit us;TO SHINE UPON THOSE WHO SIT IN DARKNESS AND THE SHADOW OF DEATH, To guide our feet into the way of peace." **Luke 78-79***

```
Dads glad he sold his car---now he won't have a
problem with all the people that were hitting him
when he drove!!!!!!!!!!..
```

There is no question this is my favorite part of the book. For years I have been intrigued by what the mind can do; especially once it is trained to work with focused intent.

Brain health is something that should be taught in school. Not necessarily the *why* about brain health, but how to accomplish and maximize its health. In this chapter I plan on providing you with ways (and resources) to stimulate your bain on a daily basis.

Before I cover games and other helpful tools, let us talk about the functions of your brain.

The Three Parts of your Brain

The human brain is made of three primary parts:

1. *The cerebrum* – This part of your brain takes up most of the space in your skull. Its functions include: problem solving, remembering, movement, feelings and thinking.

2. *The cerebellum* – This part of your brain is located under your cerebrum, at the back of your head. Its primary function is to control balance and coordination.

3. *The brain stem* – This part of the brain also resides underneath your cerebrum, in front of your cerebellum. It connects the brain and the spinal cord. Its primary function controls digestion, breathing, blood pressure and heart rate.

How Your Brain is Nourished

It is not hard to imagine how your brain is powered by your heart. Every time your heart beats blood vessels are pumped through the body to help nourish your brain. Up to 25 percent of your blood gets carried to your brain through arteries.

Once the blood reaches your brain, billions of brain cells use around 20 percent of the fuel and oxygen from your blood.

Every time you start to focus on something with intent, your brain could use up to half of that fuel and oxygen. The entire process is done through your bodies capillaries, veins, and arteries.

The Outer Layer - Cortex

Have you ever wondered why the brain looks wrinkled in pictures or diagrams? This wrinkled part of the brain is a special layer residing outside the cerebrum called the cerebral cortex. Scientists have determined certain regions of the cortex performs the following functions:

- Gives meaning of sensations from your body (things you touch), sights, sounds and smells from the outside world

- Solves problems, make plans, and generates thoughts

- Forms and stores memories

- Controls intended movement

Lefty/Righty

Though science continues to study how the left side and right side of your brain work independently, they have provided us with the following:

- *The left half* of your cerebral cortex controls everything on the right side of your body. For the most part right-handed people (those with a stronger LEFT hemisphere) are better at sequential and logical tasks. It is responsible for logic, numbers, words & writing, lists, analysis, reasoning, science & math, sequences, and linearity (single dimension).

- *The right half* of your cerebral cortex controls everything on the left side of your body. Left-handed people (those with a stronger RIGHT hemisphere) are better at creative and spatial tasks. It is also responsible for color, rhythm, imagination (creativity), art awareness, music awareness, daydreaming, holistic awareness, intuition, insight, and 3-D forms.

So how do the two halves communicate?

There is a thick band of nerve fibres called corpus callosum connecting the brain cells in both the left and right halves. Each half stays in continuous communication through these nerve fibers.

The Alzheimer Brain

Once Alzheimer's begins to run its destructive course, nerve cells begin to die. Without proper stimulation there is no chance at building new cells. Over time your brain starts to discolor due to its basically dying off cell population.

As the disease progresses your brain begins to shrink and does so dramatically. This in turn will start to affect all brain functions. Hence the warning signs I spoke on back in chapter 3.

In the case of Alzheimer's, as the massive cell death occurs the cortex shrivels creating gaps in the individuals ability to think clearly, remember, and plan. Memories are lost and fluid begins to fill the brain.

This eventually causes confusion, lack of communication, leading to lashing out then withdrawal as they no longer recognize anyone or anything.

Each individual cell in your body serves a specific function. For instance, when we meet new people, acquire new skills, and have new experiences, specific activity patterns can be noticed in the brain. Even reading, listening to others speak, thinking about words, and speaking helps spark specific activity in your brain.

These are all good activities. Brain stimulation is something to practice daily; especially early in life. This helps increase your chances of preventing many sorts of dementia down the road.

In Conclusion

There are specific activities that help preserve and develop brain strength. Do not be confused about what works. The resources I provide in the next chapter are structured to help strengthen your brain. Games like Sudoku and crossword puzzles are great for Alzheimer's prevention, but do not help much with short term memory loss.

Again, taking action is the key to success. Most of these games can be played in the morning with your first cup of coffee. This is when many are their freshest.

In chapter nine I will give you ways to flex your brain muscle.

Chapter 9

Brain Stimulation Tips & Techniques

*I like nonsense, it wakes up the brain cells. Fantasy is a necessary ingredient in living, it's a way of looking at life through the wrong end of a telescope. Which is what I do, and that enables you to laugh at life's realities. -- **Dr. Seuss***

> When dad was moved to the Alzheimer's unit in the nursing home we went to visit mom for her birthday. July 25, 2014 mom is 82 today. I told mom Jim is writing a book about Alzheimer's, do you have any funny stories you'd like to tell the world? She said, "You mean like the time I had to call the aids (at the nursing home) because dad was lost and he wasn't in our room.
>
> The aids looked all over for him and found him sitting in a recliner in another person's room in the dark while she was sleeping!"
>
> Carole

If you pay attention to trends in the media then you may have noticed a lot of talk lately about ways to stimulate your brain. There is a reason for this, though it may not be currently apparent.

Brain games like Lumosity are innovators when it comes to brain stimulation. Now keep in mind I don't have ANY association with the company. What I do know, they have one of the best programs to stimulate your brain in different ways, which can in turn lower your risk of Alzheimer's.

Remember the name of the game is to stimulate your brain to help it grow.

I'll cover just a few of the endless games you can play to increase your memory, mental flexibility, and problem solving capabilities.

Speed Match

This game challenges your processing ability as well as your reaction time. Two signs of early Alzheimer's are your inability to process new and existing information, then how you react to it.

In this game you are presented with a series of objects. Your goal is to determine whether the current object resembled the previous one. Be prepared to have fun with this one as the clock ticks adding a little more pressure to your decision.

The key to stimulating your brain is by incorporating as many processes as possible such as sight and sound. Your goal is to try and beat your score. It can become extremely addicting – in a good way.

Color Match

This game challenges your flexibility and processing speed. This is great for avoiding errors, controlling impulse, and creative problem solving.

In this game you are given two rectangle boxes each containing a color spelled out in word form. The first box has the word meaning and the second box is for color. The word in the "meaning" box describes what color the word in the "color" box should be.

Example: The words "red" and "yellow" will appear. As long as the word in the "color" box is in a yellow font, then you click "Match." If not then you click "Not a Match."

You have to react quickly and decisively. This game is a little more difficult than speed match and is scored by reaction time, accuracy and total number you get correct.

You will definitely get a mental workout in with this game.

Word Bubbles

This game exercises your language skills and flexibility. You will also work on tip-of-the-tongue and word-finding capabilities along with thinking outside of the box.

In this game you are given a word where you are to come up with as many words that start with what you are given. **Example:** "cal." You are to come up with as many words (and variations of words) starting with "cal."

This too is addicting.

Lost in Migration

This game exercises your ability to focus by avoiding distractions. This game has several benefits as it can help increase work productivity and concentration.

In this game you are given five objects (in this specific game they were birds). The birds where place in different shapes ranging from straight lines to diamonds. Your goal is to find the bird facing a different direction than the rest. You then tap the arrow getting all the birds to travel in the same direction.

You are scored by accuracy, reaction time, and total number correct.

Memory Matrix

This game really challenges your spatial recall and working memory. It's best for learning and reasoning, remembering location of objects and recalling visual patterns.

In this game you are given a set number of tiles. The game shows you colored tiles displaying specific patterns. Once the pattern is removed, you are to click on the tiles to copy the pattern. Each time you do this successfully, you are given more tiles with new patterns.

The better you get the more difficult it becomes.

Other Games

If you do a simple internet search using the keywords "Brain Games," you will find a lifetime's worth of workouts for your brain. You want to keep it simple though. It is extremely easy to get lost on the internet looking for ways to increase your mental strength.

Minutes can turn into hours and the next thing you know there is no time for anything proving to be productive. Stay disciplined by staying on the first page of whatever search engine you use. I can guanratee you will find more than enough there to keep you mentally sharp for the rest of your life.

I found a great online resource on the AARP website.

At the time of this writing, I found eight different games titled: Shapes and Colors, Split Words, Writing in the Stars, Entangled Figures, The Squeaking Mouse, Countdown, The Right Word and Private Eye.

I did not try them all, but the one I did (Countdown) was extremely challenging.

For The Non Tech-Geek

Sometimes it's nice to sit down and accomplish a goal without the need of technology. Here, I'm going to give you ways to flex your mental muscle with items everyone has or can get their hands on.

1. *Board Games*- Just about every game imaginable will fit into this category. Chess, checkers, backgammon, Candyland, etc. causes you to create strategy as well as socialize with your opponent.

2. *Jigsaw puzzles* – From personal experience this can be a double-edged sword. Only because these seem to cause more stress for me than challenging my mental capacity. However, for others, this could prove to help them stay mentally sharp.

People who are in the more advanced stages of Alzheimer's will do better with larger pieced puzzles.

3. *Cards* – Card games fit right with board games in regards to their social element. There is a great memory game where you can use 9-12 cards – all of the same suit. Place all the cards face down so they are lined up in a square three wide and three down (if using 9 cards). Make sure the cards are out of order. Flip over one card at a time to reveal its face, then flip it back over. Do this with every card. Once you do this to each card, attempt to flip the cards over again in numerical order. **Example:** Ace is 1, then find the 2...3...4, etc. This can be a fun game for the entire family.

4. *Photos, Scrapbooking & Memory Boxes* – Each of these can hold a very special place in our hearts. Each one of these three allow you to sit back and day dream about memories past. Performing these activities with others heightens the benefits.

5. *Pen & Paper* – I am a firm believer that every one of us has a story inside. It doesn't matter if you are a writer, or can even write for that matter. The key here is to release what is in your head onto something you can physically see and hold. Memories will last forever when you practice this.

6. *Idea Journal* – I wish I could take the credit for this one. In my constant drive to learn I found a podcast radio show done by James Altucher. (Matter of fact listening to two other of his shows gave me the drive to write and self-publish this exact book.) James had started to keep an idea journal where he was to write at least 10 ideas down EVERYDAY. No matter how trivial or how bad they were, he had to write down 10. In his words numbers 5-10 made him sweat and really worked what he

calls the "Idea Muscle." I now practice this and life has started to drastically turn for the better.

In Conclusion

Now I could write another entire book based on ways to help you improve your mental capacity, but I've put together a lot of information for you to digest in a short period of time. The bottom line is to simply take some type of action. This will prove to stimulate your brain keeping it strong for a lifetime.

Chapter 10

Putting It All Together

"You can talk with someone for years, everyday, and still, it won't mean as much as what you can have when you sit in front of someone, not saying a word, yet you feel that person with your heart, you feel like you have known the person for forever.... connections are made with the heart, not the tongue."

> 11/2/11 I called and asked, "What ya doing?"
>
> Dad said, "Watching mother get undresses."
>
> I said, "Hey be nice!"
>
> He says, "Gotta get her undressed before I can do anything."

One thing is for certain, in all my research a majority of the articles, websites, and books would be quick to state nothing yet guarantees to prevent Alzheimer's.

However, in my 30+ years in health and fitness, a higher percentage of the diseases running their course through people can be prevented (and some even reversed) through simple lifestyle changes. There is a common thread running through every health issue I researched, and it looks like: high cholesterol, high blood pressure, stress, and diabetes can all attribute to the development of Alzheimer's.

For a majority of people, each of those issues can be controlled with lifestyle changes - both physical and nutritionally.

Below you will find other lifestyle changes you can make to help in preventing Alzheimer's:

- Stimulate your brain muscle. Participating in mentally challenging activities (such as learning new languages or working crossword puzzles) can help reduce your chances of developing Alzheimer's disease.

- Flex your body muscle. The name of the game here is increasing blood flow. Developing lean muscle, increasing work capacity is only a couple of benefits from exercising (or participates in regular physical activity). Exercise that is of moderate intensity will help uphold cognitive function.

- Stay a Social Butterfly. In a recent longevity study, seniors living in a Nevada community had one of the lowest percentages of Alzheimer cases. The one thing that set these folks apart was their constant social interaction with each other. Being around friends is one of the best strategies a person can do to help keep Alzheimer's out of arms reach. Doing this every day helps keep the mind sharp as you are engaging in conversations with others in the community. This helps keep you mind active as you communicate with each other as well as listen to others communicate.

- Protect your heart and brain with food. Nothing is set in stone in regards to nutrition and Alzheimer's. However, the same nutrition practices that deter and reverse many of the inflammatory diseases of today is the same one that will help keep you away from Alzheimer's. Replace trans-fatty acids with saturated fats (from coconut oil) and fats from fish and plant oils. Omega-3 fatty acids (from fish oils) that contain docosahexaenoic acid (DHA) and eicosapentaenoic acid (EPA) are a necessity in your nutrition for ALL around optimum health. A diet rich in vegetable and fruit (notice how I mentioned vegetables first) will provide you with vitamins, antioxidants and other nutrients to help prevent inflammation in the body. The more colorful the more beneficial.

- Keep off the extra weight. If you are familiar with the definition of insanity then you'll understand where I am going here. Obesity is a vicious cycle that can contribute to Alzheimer's. Many people try the same gimmicks over and over to lose weight hoping - if not praying - for a different result. Obesity gives way to a sedentary lifestyle, which in-turn gives way to less activity. Eventually, you become one of the walking diseased. Your body becomes a living time-bomb riddled with inflammation and toxicity. This is like asking for diabetes, heart issues, Alzheimer's, and cancer.

Final Thoughts

Food, exercise, brain stimulation, and staying socially active are the key pillars in Alzheimer's prevention. If I could analyze these aspects of person's life, chances are they would be doing a pretty good job with Alzheimer prevention once they kept focused on them.

Over the years the one thing I've noticed is people are not off by much. Normally it is a bad habit or two that will cause those life threatening issues later down the road. Though all of these changes can seem overwhelming, and can be intimidating, this is a life-changing book.

The first step is always the hardest. However, once that first step is taken, each step after gets incrementally easier – and more beneficial.

By controlling your own vascular risk factors such as; your blood sugar, your weight, your blood pressure, and engaging in exercise, brain stimulation, and staying active, you decrease your risk of developing Alzheimer's

As of now there is no cure and the treatments are very poor. Medical professionals understand more emphasis needs to be put on prevention of this disease. If we continue at our current pace, Alzheimer's (as well as other forms of dementia) with turn into a tsunami of disease. This in turn will bankrupt our healthcare.

Easy Action Checklist

In all my years of working with people, I understand many work best with checklists. When you take the time and follow this path I laid out for you, your overall health will begin to improve immediately. But you must take that first step.

1. Nutrition – Balance is crucial. <u>Have each of these three at every meal.</u>

- **Carbohydrates** – A good rule of thumb to understand is carbohydrates make you feel hungry. The processed types will leave you looking for more within 30-60 minutes of eating them. However, each time you sit down to eat a meal (or snack), grab some vegetables and fruit. The more colorful the better. *Vegetable examples*: peppers, sweet potato, spinach, romaine lettuce, cucumber, kale, asparagus, broccoli, onion, tomato, celery, cabbage, etc. *Fruit examples:* blueberries, raspberries, blackberries, apples, strawberries, peaches, pears, etc.

- **Protein** – Just because a food label says there is protein in the food does not mean it is the correct type of protein. You need protein having a complete amino acid chain allowing lean muscle development. Lean muscle plus high metabolism equals your fat burning all day long. Here are some great *protein examples:* eggs, free-range chicken, grass-fed beef, wild-caught fish, turkey, pork, etc. Make sure your protein size is equal to the size and width of your palm.

- **Fat** – Not all fat is created equal. *Fat examples:* coconut oil, olive oil (for dressings and toppings), nuts, seeds, black olives, coconut milk, avocados, etc. are all great examples of essential fats. Don't be afraid of fat. Fat does not make you fat.

2. Exercise – Get moving! Do not make it hard, simply get active.

- **3 X 5 times a week** – Go back to chapter 6 and look over the exercise examples I gave you. Mix them up, do them for different durations, and just be creative.

- **Run, jump, play** - Play a sport, go for a walk, or go climb something. Get your heart rate up by doing something you enjoy to do. This way you will stick with it.

- **Bring a friend** – There is an old adage, *"Misery loves company."* If you find exercising miserable, get a friend involved with you. This will help keep your mind off being miserable and intimidated.

3. Flex You Brain Muscle – Challenge & stimulate your brain daily.

- **Lumosity** – In my opinion, this is one of the best tools to stimulate your brain decreasing your chances of developing Alzheimer's. Be careful because it can be addicting.

- **Puzzles & Scrapbooks** - Stimulate your brain by working on puzzles that challenge your thinking and focus. Scrapbook will help you activate memories and will bring a smile to your face.

- **Idea Journal** – Capturing your ideas on paper is the best way for you to keep your brain active in thinking of new things. Writing down at least 10 ideas a day will keep your thinking sharp. And who knows, you may have an idea to help change the world…I did which led to this book.

Chapter 11

Life Stories: Why You Should Be Journaling Now

"These handwritten words in the pages of my journal confirm that from an early age I have experienced each encounter in my life twice: once in the world, and once again on the page." --**Terry Tempest Williams**

> "Get me my aftershave drink, I am out!"
>
> "Huh?" Now I thought he drank his Aqua Velva! I say, "What are you talking about?"
>
> He says, "You know, the colored stuff in the fridge...THAT I DRINK AFTER I SHAVE."

The one thing that can be disappointing is the number of people who've lived great lives and then fall by the way side – lost forever when they pass on to the next life. Far too many people brush off the power of journaling for whatever reason. When in all actuality the exact opposite is the case...

...everyone should be journaling.

So many stories go untold, left as a distant memory. Only the few stories told by family members and friends who end up remembering only a portion of what really happened.

I will be honest and tell you I've not given it much thought until recently. I can remember when and why this hit me like a ton of bricks.

It was when Carole and I sat down and watched the movie, "The Notebook."

Ten years after the movie came out (fourteen years after the novel was published) I finally decided to watch the movie. I had no clue as to what the movie was about and found myself speechless as I watched it: Drawn in like no other movie had drawn me in.

Carole and I joke on occasion that we should have journaled *"our"* story. As of yet we have not done it.

The Notebook really opened my eyes to the world of dementia. Now that it is in the family I can see the effects of the disease firsthand. It can be an extremely painful event for everyone involved.

Imagine what life would be like if you one day forgot your personal story – or that of a loved one. This is why I've taken upon myself to help people write their life stories (otherwise known as memoirs).

I've always been a firm believer that the foundation of our country was laid by our seniors. Instead of learning generalized history in school from history books, think of what it would be like if every family had a memoir to pass down from generation to generation.

Just like many people are intrigued by their family genealogy, family life stories would last the test of time.

One of the best and easiest ways to get started here is by scrap booking. Old pictures, souvenirs, and other treasured items make great tools to jar your memory. Going through boxes stuffed in the attic, garage, and even a shed could prove to be a goldmine of memories. On a Sunday morning while you're drinking your favorite morning drink, grab your memory box, scrapbook, or whatever, and just start to write.

Write with total abandonment. Don't worry about anything making sense. Most of us think faster than we write. Stopping to self-edit every time you notice something wrong is frustrating.

Once you get frustrated you will be more apt to quit. Then all will be lost and chances are you won't give it another shot.

Honestly, journaling can be one of the best defenses against Alzheimer's. It helps you relive all the great things that happened over the course of your life.

If you find writing your life story a daunting task, seeking help could be the easiest way to get your story down where it will never be forgotten. This is where I may be able to help you.

I can help you get your life story down once you are ready to start your own life history book. The key is to interview the important people in your life who make your story unique. This is an easy task. I use specific questions to help pull out all the hidden nuggets to making your story become a page-turner.

Don't let your life pass you by and become a distant family memory. Shoot me an email at: jim@JimTurnboHealth.com.

Once you have your key memories in your head, your story will begin to write itself.

If you want to keep up to date on the most recent news about Alzheimer's and to get access to the first two chapters of my book "Beating Alzheimer's Through Nutrition – What You Eat Today Determines Your Life Tomorrow," simply visit me at: http://JimTurnboHealth.com.

About the Author

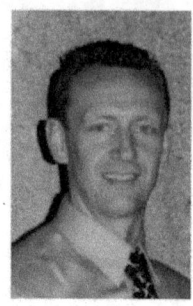

Over the last three decades, Jim Turnbo III has spent thousands of hours and thousands of dollars traveling to gyms all over the world. Each stint only developed frustration with "routines," people and the lack of results. Not until 7 years ago did he finally start to stumble across the answers to his most pressing health and fitness questions.

These same questions continue to rear their ugly heads over and over in the lives of the people he comes across.

Can he say ALL his questions have been answered? Not Even Close!!!

The one answer he did develop was this – health, exercise, nutrition, longevity….is an evolution. It's in a state of constant change. More importantly it's a lifestyle.

"I've tried just about every supplement, program, fad diet/exercise program…you name it. I tried them all!" says Turnbo.

This life-long evolution has brought him to where he is now.

No one workout program is perfect for everyone. One eating lifestyle may work for one, but won't work for many more. It all comes down to what your goals and needs are. Some may get all the nutrients they need from the food they consume, however a bigger

> *"It's virtually impossible for the normal person to figure out everything they need - for optimal health - from all the different diets, fads and gimmicks in existence today; especially when they are constantly conflicting."*

percentage of us need to supplement in some capacity.

Whether its weight loss/management, energy or athletic improvement, we need to have the best tools available.

Jim's intention was to help guide you down the path of optimal health. This path can be one of the most confusing roads you will have to travel today. With all the options available, it gets EXTREMELY hard to sift through the hype, false promises and the myths portrayed by the "experts."

It wasn't until recently did he really hone in on his God given call in life. Some of you call it your gift or what you do for a living. For Jim, it is the code he lives by and it stems from Isaiah 30:21

"Whether you turn to the right or to the left, your ears will hear a voice behind you, saying, "This is the way; walk in it."

We all fall off the path in life. That is inevitable! It's not until someone reminds us how to get back on the right path, do we realize it. With that guidance, I can GUARANTEE you will achieve whatever you have your heart set on.

Continue to move forward...

Your Next Step

- Check out many of his articles on exercise, nutrition, and the spiritual side of life on his blog at: www.JimTurnboHealth.com.

  Make sure you sign up for his newsletters for health tips to take your life to the next level

- Let's meet face to face on Facebook. Simply cut and paste the below link, like my page and we will get to know each other:

  www.facebook.com/jimturnbohealth

Other Books by Jim Turnbo III

"Beating Alzheimer's: *Life Altering Tips To Help Prevent You From Becoming Another Statistic*"

"*50 Ways To Stimulate Your Brain: Simple Tips To Keep Your Brain Healthy and Strong For A Lifetime*"

www.ingramcontent.com/pod-product-compliance
Lightning Source LLC
Chambersburg PA
CBHW060153290526
45789CB00003B/1027